PEAK PERFORMANCE

THE NEW
GLUCOSE
revolution

Other books in the New Glucose Revolution Series

PEAK PERFORMANCE

THE NEW
GLUCOSE
revolution

HELEN O'CONNOR
PROF JENNIE BRAND-MILLER
PROF STEPHEN COLAGIURI
KAYE FOSTER-POWELL

HODDER

A Hodder Book

First published in Australia and New Zealand in 1998
by Hodder Headline Australia Pty Limited
(A member of the Hodder Headline Group)
Level 22, 201 Kent Street, Sydney NSW 2000

Website: www.hha.com.au

Reprinted 1999, 2000

This edition published as *The New Glucose Revolution Peak Performance* in 2003

National Library of Australia
Cataloguing-in-Publication data

The new glucose revolution peak performance.

Rev. ed.
ISBN 0 7336 1708 5.

1. Athletes - Nutrition. 2. Glycemic index. 3. Food - Carbohydrate content. I. Brand-Miller, Jennie, 1952- .
II. Title : The G.I. factor : the glucose revolution : sports nutrition.

613.2024796

Cover by Greendot Design
Cover image © photolibrary. com
Typeset by Egan-Reid Ltd, Auckland
Printed in Australia by Griffin Press, Adelaide

CONTENTS

INTRODUCTION

What you eat does make a difference to your performance. Australian scientists were the first in the world to apply the concept of the glycemic index to sport and exercise science. It may be no coincidence that Australians are famed for their sporting prowess around the world. They have been world champions in swimming, cricket, tennis, rugby and netball year after year.

The trick is getting into the right eating routine, keeping up to date and ignoring the confusing nutrition myths that abound. Understanding the GI and how to apply this to your diet can give you the winning edge—whether you are one of the elite or a weekend warrior.

As we explain in our bestselling book, *The New Glucose Revolution*, the glycemic index:

- is a scientifically proven measure of the effect carbohydrates have on blood glucose levels
- helps you choose the right type of carbohydrate for your health and wellbeing
- provides an easy and effective way to eat a healthy diet and control fluctuations in blood glucose.

In this book we will show you how the GI can help you choose the right foods to reach your maximum potential in sporting events.

For more detailed information about the glycemic index and its many benefits you should consult *The New Glucose Revolution* or *The New Glucose Revolution Life Plan* which provides even more recipes and practical information.

WHAT THIS BOOK CAN DO FOR YOU

The GI ranks carbohydrates in foods according to their glycemic impact. The rise in blood glucose affects the insulin response to that food and ultimately affects the fuel mix and carbohydrate stores available to the exercising muscles. In sport and exercise, there may be times when some individuals will benefit from choosing low GI foods (e.g. *before* the event) and times when high GI foods are better (e.g. *during* and *after* the event). For best performance, a serious athlete needs to learn about which foods have high and low GI values and when to eat them.

But it's not only the type of carbohydrate that matters—the amount of carbohydrate is equally important. Training diets must provide adequate carbohydrate if the GI is to make any difference at all.

When you pop this pocket book into your training bag, you'll have:

- a quick quiz to help you assess your current eating habits
- refuelling hints at your fingertips
- case studies that provide you with fun, easy and practical ways to eat your way to better performance
- the GI values of over 400 foods, including sports drinks

What you eat does make a difference to your sports performance.

IS YOUR DIET FIT FOR PEAK PERFORMANCE?

Take the diet fitness quiz and see how well you score. It's a good idea to use this quiz regularly to pick up on areas where you may need to improve your diet.

Circle your answer.

Eating patterns

☐ I eat at least 3 meals a day with no longer than 5 hours in between
Yes/No

Carbohydrate checker

☐ I eat at least 4 slices of bread (or alternatives) each day (2 slices of bread = ½ cup rice, 1 potato)
Yes/No

☐ I eat at least 1 cup breakfast cereal each day or an extra slice of bread
Yes/No

☐ I usually eat 2 or more pieces of fruit each day
Yes/No

I eat at least 3 different vegetables or have a salad most days
Yes/No

☐ I include carbohydrates like pasta, rice and potato in my diet each day
Yes/No

Protein checker

☐ I eat at least 1 and usually 2 serves of meat or meat alternatives (poultry, seafood, eggs, dried peas/beans or nuts) each day
Yes/No

Calcium checker

☐ I eat at least 3 serves of dairy food or calcium—fortified soy milk alternative each day (1 serve = 200 ml milk or fortified soy milk; 1 slice (30 g) hard cheese; 200 g yoghurt)
Yes/No

Fat checker

☐ I spread butter or margarine thinly on bread or use
none at all
Yes/No

☐ I eat deep fried food no more than once per week
Yes/No

☐ I use modest amounts of polyunsaturated or monounsaturated oil (Canola or olive) for cooking
Yes/No

☐ I avoid oil-based dressings on salads
Yes/No

☐ I use reduced fat or low fat dairy products
Yes/No

☐ I cut the fat off meat and take the skin off chicken
Yes/No

☐ I eat fatty snacks such as chocolate, chips, biscuits,
rich desserts, cakes, pies and pastries no more than
twice per week
Yes/No

☐ I eat fast or take-away food no more than once per
week
Yes/No

Iron checker

☐ I eat lean red meat at least 3 times per week or 2 servings of white meat daily or for vegetarians, include at least 1–2 cups of dried peas and beans (e.g. lentils, soy beans, chick peas) daily
Yes/No

☐ I include a vitamin C source with meals based on bread, cereals, fruit and vegetables to assist the iron absorption in these 'plant' sources of iron
Yes/No

Fluids

☐ I drink fluids regularly before, during and after exercise
Yes/No

Alcohol

☐ I usually have at least 2 alcohol free days per week and do not drink more than two standard drinks★ (for women) or four standard drinks★ (for men) on other days
Yes/No
(Circle yes if you don't drink more alcohol)

Score I point for every 'yes' answer	
Scoring scale	
18–20 Excellent	15–17 Room for improvement
12–14 Just made it	0–12 Poor

Note: Very active people will need to eat more breads, cereals and fruit than on this quiz, but to stay healthy no one should be eating less.

The amounts of foods in this quiz are devised for adults NOT children or adolescents

★ Standard drink:
- 1 middy (285 mls) of regular beer
- 1 schooner (425 mls) of light or low alcohol beer
- 1 nip of spirits
- 100 ml of wine

(Adapted from *The Taste of Fitness* by Helen O'Connor and Donna Hay)

YOUR GUIDE TO SPORTS NUTRITION

High carbohydrate eating

To perform at its best, your body needs the right type of fuel. No matter what your sport, carbohydrates are an important fuel. High carbohydrate foods help enhance stamina and prevent fatigue. They include, breakfast cereals, bread, rice, pasta, fruit and vegetables (especially starchy vegetables like potato, corn and dried peas and beans). Sugars found in table sugar, honey, jam and confectionery are also useful sources of carbohydrate for active people. See pages 20–5 for more information about carbohydrates.

Low fat eating

Fats are an essential part of your diet. A low to moderate fat intake helps active people maintain a lean physique. Eating the best types of fat and avoiding excessive fat intake is important for good health and peak performance. The best types of fats for cooking include monounsaturated fats like olive and canola oil and polyunsaturated fats like sunflower and safflower oil. Watch out for the saturated fats found in many fast foods, butter, cream and the fat on meat.

Fat reducing strategies include:

- cutting the fat off meat (or using trim cuts)
- removing the skin from chicken
- using minimal amounts of fat in cooking
- using non-stick cookware

The amount of fat you need depends on your daily fuel requirements. For good health and weight maintenance we have included the following general guidelines. (Note: 5 grams of fat is equivalent to about 1 teaspoon mono- or polyunsaturated oil.)

Low fat diets	30–40 g fat per day
Most women and children	30–50 g fat per day
Most men	40–60 g fat per day
Teenagers and active adults	70 g fat per day
Larger and very active athletes/workers	80–100 g fat per day

Fat is an 'invisible' ingredient in many foods. Use a fat counter to help you identify some of the sources of fat in your diet. Keep a food record for a week and calculate your personal fat intake using the counter. It may surprise you! Comprehensive fat counters are readily available from bookshops and newsagents.

Don't forget protein

Athletes in heavy training have increased protein needs. Protein balance depends on the individual but you generally need at least 2 servings a day. Some athletes forget to include enough protein in their diet (2–3 serves per day). Body building athletes often consume protein in excess of their requirements. Good sources of protein include lean meat, poultry, fish and seafood, eggs, milk, cheese and yoghurt. Dried peas, beans and nuts are the best vegetable source. Bread and cereals provide smaller but still useful amounts of protein.

Fluids

The human body is 70 per cent water. During exercise you lose some of this water as sweat. If you don't replace it, you will become dehydrated and your body will overheat—like a car without water in its radiator.

- Small fluid losses decrease mental and physical performance.
- Large fluid losses resulting in dehydration are life threatening!

During exercise, thirst is not a good indicator of your fluid needs. You usually need to drink more than your thirst dictates. Every kilogram lost during exercise approximates 1 litre of sweat losses to be replaced.

> **During exercise,
> thirst is not a good indicator
> of your fluid needs.**

What to drink during exercise

Water is an adequate fluid replacer and is appropriate in many situations.

Sports or electrolyte replacement drinks are absorbed into the blood stream faster than water, replace carbohydrates and electrolytes, and have a pleasant taste—which encourages greater fluid consumption. See pages 54–57 for more on sports drinks. The tables at the back of the book give the GI of sports drinks, such as Gatorade.

Please note that this does not refer to sport supplement drinks like Sustagen Sport, which is a liquid meal rather than an electrolyte replacer.

Soft drinks or fruit juice empty from the stomach slower than sports/electrolyte drinks or water and aren't suitable fluid replacers during exercise.

Adequate fluid replacement during exercise enhances performance and prevents heat stress.

Iron

Iron deficiency is common in athletes, particularly female athletes, vegetarians, and those participating in strenuous training programs, especially endurance athletes. Many athletes don't consume adequate iron in their daily diet and may include excess caffeine or tannin (in tea) that binds up iron and reduces its absorption. The richest sources of iron are red meats, liver and kidney. Plant sources contain lower amounts of iron which is not absorbed as well. The iron in iron supplements is also less well absorbed than the iron in red meat.

Sources of iron (ranked from best to least):

* * * *	Red meats, liver, kidney
* * *	White meats and seafood
* *	Dried peas and beans (baked beans, soy beans)
*	Bread, iron-enriched breakfast cereals and some vegetables

Did you know?

Including vitamin C rich fruits and vegetables in a meal improves the absorption of iron from plant sources (e.g. bread, cereals, vegetables, fruit). Drinking a glass of orange juice with your cereal in the morning will increase the amount of iron absorbed from this meal.

Calcium

Calcium is important for bone development in the young and for bone maintenance in adults. An adequate calcium intake and weight-bearing exercise throughout life is essential to build and then maintain optimal bone strength for both males and females.

> **Calcium is important
> for bone development in the young
> and for bone maintenance in adults.**

In females, regular strenuous exercise, usually accompanied by factors such as fat loss, strict dieting or stress, can precipitate menstrual cycle interruptions. An irregular or absent menstrual cycle may result in a reduced level of the hormone oestrogen which is vital for maintaining calcium levels in bone and for enhancing calcium absorption from the diet. Menstrual irregularities of greater than six months need medical investigation. Athletes with very infrequent or absent menstrual cycles should have extra calcium in the range of 1000 to 1500 milligrams a day. This won't prevent bone loss but may help to slow down the rate of loss.

Nutritional supplements

Big dollars are spent promoting nutritional supplements for active people and athletes. Watch out for supplements with no scientific basis to the claims. If in doubt, ask a sports dietitian for help. Some supplements are beneficial in certain circumstances.

Supplements of iron or calcium may be required if inadequate amounts are consumed in the diet or if deficiency exists.

Supplements like sports drinks, liquid meals and carbohydrate loaders are also beneficial, not because they provide something magical but because they package energy and carbohydrate in a convenient and easy to consume form. This is especially useful to athletes who need an easily digested fuel on the run.

Sports bars and carbohydrate gels (available in sports and bike shops) are in a similar category to sports drinks etc.

Herbal supplements, amino acids and fat burners. Unfortunately, solid evidence for these supplements is lacking. In many cases, scientific studies have shown they have absolutely no effect on fat loss, muscle growth or performance.

Did you know?

Elite and professional athletes need to check all their medications and supplements with the Australian Sports Drug Agency (ASDA) prior to taking. Some dietary supplements are on the "banned" list as they can cause a positive drug test and result in disqualification and sanctions which may prevent the athlete from competing for a designated period.

THE IMPORTANCE OF CARBOHYDRATE

Carbohydrate circulates in your body as glucose in the blood (blood sugar) and is stored as glycogen in the liver and muscles. Your body uses glucose to fuel movement and activity. Just as high speed cars require regular top-ups of petrol, active bodies need a regular supply of carbohydrate to maintain adequate glycogen stores. When glycogen stores are depleted, fatigue sets in and performance suffers.

Carbohydrate is the human body's main
energy source for physical activity,
especially high intensity exercise.

Your body's carbohydrate stores are small and need regular replenishing, generally every 4 to 5 hours. Athletes feel tired and lethargic when they don't consume enough carbohydrate for their daily needs. When this happens and the glycogen in the muscles is depleted, fatigue sets in. That's when your muscles feel heavy and your pace slows. 'Hitting the wall', an expression used by endurance athletes, refers to the feeling when glycogen stores are almost exhausted.

Low blood sugar or 'hypoglycemia'

Exercisers can also experience a type of fatigue related to the carbohydrate levels in their blood. It is possible for your muscle glycogen levels to be adequate while the blood glucose levels, controlled by the liver, fall. Low blood glucose or 'hypoglycaemia' (cyclists call this 'bonking') usually occurs when you exercise in the morning before eating, or exercise hard after skipping a meal.

Early morning exercise

If you exercise strenuously early in the morning, it's a good idea to have some carbohydrate before training or take some with you to have on the run! Most people have enough liver glycogen to fuel low intensity, short duration (i.e. less than 1 hour) exercise sessions. If you simply want to delay eating until after your light early morning walk, it's not a problem. However, eating before and/or during a strenuous cycling session makes good sense!

> To maintain energy levels,
> athletes must consume enough carbohydrate
> on a regular basis to keep pace with their
> muscle glycogen needs and maintain normal
> blood glucose levels.

Carbohydrate

Carbohydrate mainly comes from plant foods, such as cereal grains, fruits, vegetables and legumes (peas and beans). Milk products also contain carbohydrate in the form of milk sugar or lactose. Lactose is the first carbohydrate we encounter as infants and human milk lactose is higher in lactose than any other mammal milk. It accounts for almost half the energy available to the infant. Some foods contain a large amount of carbohydrate (such as cereals, potatoes and legumes) while other foods are very dilute sources (such as carrots, broccoli and salad vegetables). So, as nutritious as a salad with lettuce, tomatoes, carrots, egg and celery etc. is, it isn't a meal on its own and needs to be complemented with a carbohydrate food like wholegrain bread or pasta.

Foods that are high in carbohydrate:

Cereal grains including rice, wheat, oats, barley, rye and anything made from them (bread, pasta, noodles, flour, breakfast cereal).

Fruit

Vegetables such as potatoes, yams, sweet corn, taro and sweet potato.

Legumes including baked beans, lentils, kidney beans and chickpeas.

Dairy products such as yoghurt and ice-cream.

Sources of carbohydrate

Percentage of carbohydrate (grams per 100 grams of food) in food as eaten

milk 5%	split peas 45%
plum 6%	bread 47%
peas 8%	oats 61%
orange 8%	barley 61%
baked beans 11%	wheat biscuit 62%
apple 12%	pasta 70%
pear 12%	water cracker 71%
grapes 15%	flour 73%
potato 15%	sultanas 75%
sweet corn 16%	rice 79%
sweet potato 17%	cornflakes 85%
banana 21%	tapioca 85%
ice-cream 22%	sugar 100%

HOW MUCH CARBOHYDRATE DO YOU NEED?

It is difficult to put an exact figure on anyone's carbohydrate needs. Use the following table as a rough guide and ask a sports dietitian for help if you are unsure.

Active bodies need a regular supply of carbohydrate to maintain adequate glycogen stores.

Three easy steps to estimate your daily carbohydrate needs

Step 1. Weigh yourself naked or in minimal clothing in kilograms;

Step 2. Multiply your body weight by your activity level (see following table). This total gives you the **target carbohydrate intake in grams** that you must consume each day to meet your carbohydrate needs.

Step 3. Keep a food record for a few days and calculate your carbohydrate intake with a carbohydrate counter such as the one at the end of this book. Compare your actual carbohydrate intake with the target value you calculated. If it is way below the carbohydrate target, you have some serious carb eating to do! If you are within 50 grams or even a little over your carbohydrate target that's fine. Use the carbohydrate counter to help you plan an adequate carbohydrate intake.

Remember, this is a rough estimate.
You may need a little more or less.
See how you feel.

What's your activity level?

The amount of carbohydrate you need depends on your weight and activity level.

Activity Level		Grams of carbohydrate per kg body weight per day
Light	Walking, light/easy swimming or cycling, low impact/easy beat aerobic dance	4–5
Less than 1 hour per day		
Light-moderate	intermediate aerobic dance class, easy jog, non-competitive tennis (3 sets), netball	5–6
1 hour per day		
Moderate	1 hour run, serious training for recreational/ competition sports such as soccer, basketball, squash	6–7
1–2 hours per day		

Activity Level		Grams of carbohydrate per kg body weight per day
Moderate-heavy	most professional/elite training for competitive sport such as swimming, tennis, football, distance running (marathon)	7–8
2–4 hours per day		
Heavy	Training for ironman events marathon running/ swimming, Ironman triathlon	8–10
More than 4 hours per day		

Activity levels refer to the intensity
as well as the duration of the activity.

Time refers to the amount of time you are
physically active during training, not the
amount of time at training.

Body weight refers to ideal
or 'healthy' body weight.

Example of a carbohydrate calculation

Jessica's carbohydrate needs

Step 1.   Weight 58 kg

Step 2.   Activity—Moderate level (training for mid-distance fun runs such as City to Surf—recreational level)

Requires 6–7 g of carbohydrate per kilogram per day

Target carbohydrate level is:
$6 \times 58 = 348$ g per day to
$7 \times 58 = 406$ g per day

348–406 g per day

Step 3. Food Record

Jessica's food record

Meal		Carbohydrate count (g)
Breakfast	1 cup of bran cereal	35
	½ cup of milk	5
	1 slice of white toast with butter	15
	150ml no added sugar fruit juice	15
Snack	1 banana	32
Lunch	1 cheese and tomato sandwich on white bread	32
	1 low fat fruit yoghurt	26
	1 glass water	0
Snack	2 cracker biscuits with Vegemite™	12
	1 orange	10
Dinner	1 small piece of steak	0
	1 medium potato	16
	½ cup of mixed vegetables	7
	2 small scoops reduced fat ice-cream	13

Supper	3 plain coffee biscuits	14
Total carbohydrate		**225 g**

Jessica's carbohydrate count is way below target.
To boost Jessica's carbohydrate intake, add:

1 extra piece of toast at breakfast	15
1 extra sandwich and fruit or juice at lunch	45
1 cup cooked pasta or rice with dinner	55
1 bread roll with dinner	30
1 glass of hot milk at supper	7

Grand total boosted with the extra carbohydrate foods	**377 g**

This is in the middle of the recommended range for Jessica's weight and activity level. Depending on how she feels, slight adjustments may be required depending on variations in the intensity and duration of her training program.

Many active people, especially athletes in heavy training who eat large volumes of food, easily meet their daily nutrient requirements. Their carbohydrate needs, however, are sometimes so high, they simply can't manage the volume they need to eat! Liquid meals or carbohydrate supplements can help these athletes with high energy requirements to meet their energy needs in a less 'bulky' way.

Today, there's another consideration
in selecting carbohydrate foods
to boost your sports performance.
It is the glycemic index of a food—the GI.

UNDERSTANDING THE GI

The glycemic index concept was first developed in 1981 by Dr David Jenkins, a professor of nutrition at the University of Toronto, Canada, to help determine which foods were best for people with diabetes. At that time, the diet for people with diabetes was based on a system of carbohydrate exchanges, which assumed that all starchy foods produced the same effect on blood glucose levels, even though earlier studies had already proven this was not correct. Jenkins was one of the first people to question this assumption and investigate how real foods behave in the bodies of real people.

Since then, scientists, including the authors of this book, have tested the effect of many foods on blood glucose levels and clinical studies in the United

Kingdom, France, Italy, Australia and Canada all have proven without doubt the value of the glycemic index.

The GI of foods is simply a ranking of carbohydrates in foods according to their immediate impact on blood glucose levels. To make a fair comparison, all foods are compared with a reference food such as pure glucose and are tested in equivalent carbohydrate amounts.

Today we know the GI of hundreds of different food items that have been tested following the standardised method. We have included many of these values in the tables at the back of this book, but for more detailed information you should consult *The New Glucose Revolution* or *The New Glucose Revolution Tables*.

The key is the rate of digestion

Foods containing carbohydrates that break down quickly during digestion have the highest GI value. The blood glucose response is fast and high (in other words, the glucose in the bloodstream increases rapidly). Conversely, foods that contain carbohydrates which break down slowly, releasing glucose gradually into the bloodstream have low GI values.

For most people, the foods with a low GI have advantages over those with high GI values.

The higher the GI, the higher the blood glucose levels after consumption of the food. Instant white rice (GI 87) and baked potatoes (GI 85) have very high GIs, meaning their effect on blood glucose levels is almost as high as that of an equal amount of pure glucose (yes, you read it correctly).

Low GI = 55 or less
Intermediate GI = 56 to 69
High GI = 70 or more

Figure 1 shows the blood glucose response to potatoes compared with pure glucose. Foods with a low GI (like lentils at 29) show a flatter blood glucose response when eaten, as shown in Figure 2. The peak blood glucose level is lower and the return to baseline levels is slower than with a high GI food.

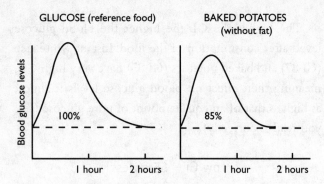

Figure 1. The effect of pure glucose (50 g) and baked potatoes without fat (50 g carbohydrate portion) on blood glucose levels.

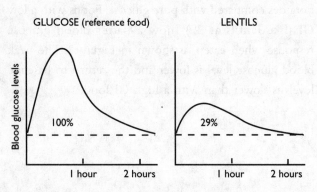

Figure 2. The effect of pure glucose (50 g) and lentils (50 g carbohydrate portion) on blood glucose levels.

How we measure the GI

Pure glucose produces the greatest rise in blood glucose levels. Most foods have less effect when fed in equal carbohydrate quantities. The GI of pure glucose is set at 100 and every other food is ranked on a scale from 1 to 100 according to its actual effect on blood glucose levels.

1. An amount of food containing a standard amount of carbohydrate (usually 25 or 50 grams) is given to a volunteer to eat. For example, to test boiled spaghetti, the volunteer will be given 200 grams of spaghetti which supplies 50 grams of carbohydrate (determined from food composition tables).

2. Over the next two hours (or three hours if the volunteer has diabetes), we take a sample of their blood every 15 minutes during the first hour and thereafter every 30 minutes. The blood glucose level of these blood samples is measured in the laboratory and recorded.

3. The blood glucose level is plotted on a graph and the area under the curve is calculated using a computer program (Figure 3).

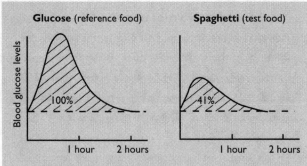

Figure 3. Measuring the GI of a food

The test food and the reference food must contain the same amount of carbohydrate. The usual dose is 50 grams but sometimes 25 grams is used when the portion size would be otherwise too large. Even smaller doses such as 15 grams have been used. The GI result is much the same whatever the dose because the GI is simply a relative measure of carbohydrate quality.

4. The volunteer's response to spaghetti (or whatever food is being tested) is compared with his or her blood glucose response to 50 grams of pure glucose (the reference food).

5. The reference food is tested on two or three separate occasions and an average value is calculated. This is done to reduce the effect of day-to-day variation in blood glucose responses.

6. The average GI found in 8–10 people is the GI of that food.

Is there an easy way to tell if a food has a high or low GI ?

No! The only way to tell is to measure the blood glucose response to that food. Generally, foods that break down quickly during digestion have the highest GI values. The GI cannot be predicted from the chemical composition of the food or the GI of related foods. Milling and grinding break down the cellular structure of grains and tend to speed up the rate of digestion, which increases the GI. Cooking increases the digestibility of starch, and may also increase the GI. It might seem surprising but removing the dietary fibre in bread, rice or pasta has little effect on the GI. However, the viscous fibre found in fruits and some grains (e.g. oats and barley) may account for their lower GI. Fat slows the digestion process and lowers the GI in some instances.

What gives one food a high GI and another a low one?

The physical state of the starch in the food is the most important factor influencing the GI. That's why food processing has such a profound effect on the GI.

Factors that influence the GI of a food

Factor	Mechanism	Examples of food where the effect is seen
Starch gelatinisation	The less gelatinised (swollen) the starch, the slower the rate of digestion.	Spaghetti, porridge, biscuits have less gelatinised starch.
Physical entrapment	The fibrous coat around beans and seeds and plant cell walls acts as a physical barrier, slowing down access of enzymes to the starch inside.	Pumpernickel and grainy bread, legumes and barley.
High amylose to amylopectin ratio*	The more amylose a food contains, the less easily the starch is gelatinised and the slower its rate of digestion.	Basmati rice, legumes, Hi-Maize™ starch contain more amylose than other cereals.
Particle size	The smaller the particle size, the easier it is for water and enzymes to penetrate (the surface area is relatively higher).	Finely milled flours have high GIs. Stone-ground flours have larger particles and lower GIs.

Factors that influence the GI of a food *(cont.)*

Factor	Mechanism	Examples of food where the effect is seen
Viscosity of fibre	Viscous, soluble fibres increase the viscosity of the intestinal contents and this slows down the interaction between the starch and the enzymes. Finely milled wholemeal wheat and rye flours have fast rates of digestion and absorption because the fibre is not viscous.	Rolled oats, beans and lentils, apples, Metamucil®.
Sugar	The digestion of sugar produces only half as many glucose molecules as the same amount of starch (the other half is fructose). The presence of sugar also restricts gelatinisation of the starch by binding water and reducing the amount of 'available' water.	Some biscuits, some breakfast cereals that are high in sugar have relatively low GI values.
Acidity	Acids in foods slow down stomach emptying, thereby slowing the rate at which the starch can be digested.	Vinegar, lemon juice, lime juice, salad dressings, pickled vegetables, sourdough bread.
Fat	Fat slows down the rate of stomach emptying, thereby slowing the digestion of the starch.	Potato crisps have a lower GI than boiled potatoes.

* Amylose and amylopectin are two different types of starch. Both are found in foods, but the ratio varies.

Tricky twins

Circle the food in each of the following pairs which you think will have the lower GI value.

Rice	Rice Bubbles
Sweet corn	Cornflakes
Baked potatoes	French fries
Toasted muesli	Untoasted muesli
Grainy bread	Wholemeal bread

(Answers: Rice (depending on the brand), Sweet corn, Baked potatoes, Toasted muesli, Grainy bread—depending on the brand.)

REACHING PEAK PERFORMANCE WITH THE GI

There are several applications of the GI to sports performance. Sometimes it will be best for you to choose a high GI food, other times some individuals may benefit from using a low GI food or meal.

To date, most work on the GI and peak performance has concentrated on the pre-event meal and competition eating and recovery.

Misconceptions about carbohydrates

Many athletes and coaches have misconceptions about carbohydrates that can affect athletic performance. In the past we were taught that simple carbohydrates (sugars) were digested and absorbed rapidly while complex carbohydrates (starches) were digested slowly. We assumed (completely incorrectly) that simple carbohydrates gave the most rapid rises in blood sugar while complex carbohydrates produced gradual rises. Unfortunately, these assumptions had no factual or scientific basis. Instead, they were based on structural considerations: smaller molecules, like sugars, were thought to be easier to digest than larger ones, such as starches. Even though incorrect, the logical nature of these assumptions meant that they were rarely ever questioned. Unfortunately, many people still think sugars are the best source of quick energy and that starches are our best source of sustained energy.

How carbohydrates can help

Scientific research has so far identified four applications of the glycemic index to enhance performance.

1. A low GI pre-event meal in some circumstances may enhance endurance in prolonged exercise.
2. High GI foods or fluids during exercise help to maintain blood glucose levels.
3. High GI foods in the recovery phase after exercise help to accelerate glycogen replenishment.
4. Low GI foods may help athletes and 'week-end warriors' alike to feel full and satisfied after and between meals and this may assist them to maintain a more optimal weight or body fat level for their sport.

Researchers at the University of Sydney in Australia found a number of years ago that a low GI pre-event meal, at least one hour prior to endurance exercise delayed fatigue by delivering greater amounts of carbohydrate to the muscle late in exercise.

Look at it this way: the low GI meal will still be digesting while you exercise and providing an additional source of carbohydrate that you had long forgotten about. Slow-release (low GI) carbohydrate is thought to be particularly useful for exercise of long duration when glycogen stores become limited. This is especially true when the ability to consume carbohydrate during the event is difficult or limited.

Low GI foods, because they are absorbed much more slowly, can be likened to a continuous injection of glucose during the event. This glucose 'infusion' can boost energy when fatigue begins to set in. Low GI pre-exercise meals also help to decrease the secretion of the hormone insulin which inhibits the body's ability to burn fat during exercise. Lower insulin levels pre-event help to promote better fat burning early in exercise and result in a 'sparing' of muscle glycogen. This 'spared' glycogen is then available for when the intensity of exercise increases or late in exercise there is still some glycogen left which will help to delay fatigue.

Eating for competing: carbohydrate loading

Carbohydrate (or glycogen) loading increases the body's store of glycogen in the liver and muscles. The extra glycogen provides additional fuel for endurance exercise where a normal glycogen store will not be sufficient to maintain stamina.

Early loading methods included a glycogen depletion phase which was employed to make the muscles 'hungry' for glycogen. These early regimes were like torture, as athletes felt tired, irritable and had difficulty maintaining motivation and concentration. After 2–3 day of the depletion phase, a high carbohydrate diet providing 9–10 grams of carbohydrate for every kilogram of body weight was consumed for a further 3 days. During this time, glycogen stores increased by 200–300 per cent.

In recent times, a modified carbohydrate loading regimen has been developed that results in a similar glycogen store without the unpleasant 'depletion' phase. Athletes simply taper training in the week prior to competition and consume a high carbohydrate diet as described above for 2–3 days prior to competition.

Do you need to carbohydrate load?

Most athletes only need an adequate normal store of carbohydrate to maximise performance. Carbohydrate loading, in its true sense, is only needed for endurance athletes exercising for greater than 120 minutes in duration, for example those competing in sports like triathlon, marathon running or ironman events.

What about the GI and carbohydrate loading?

At present there is insufficient scientific evidence to recommend a particular GI for carbohydrate loading. It appears that high GI diets may result in higher muscle glycogen levels in non-athletes. It would seem reasonable to propose that a higher GI diet may facilitate more effective glycogen loading, but further research is needed.

Carbohydrate loading increases
the body's store of glycogen.
This helps prevent fatigue
in endurance events.

BEFORE THE EVENT

Researchers at the University of Sydney several years ago found that a low GI pre-event meal, at least 1 hour prior to endurance exercise delayed fatigue by delivering greater amounts of carbohydrate to the muscle late in exercise. If you think about it, the low GI meal will still be digesting during the exercise session and providing an additional source of carbohydrate that you had long forgotten about. Slow-release (low GI) carbohydrate is thought to be particularly useful for exercise of long duration where glycogen stores usually become limiting.

Since the publication of the above research there have been a number of other studies investigating the effect of low GI pre-event meals. Some of these studies show improved exercise performance, others do not. One important issue to consider with low GI pre-event meals is whether carbohydrate will be consumed during exercise in the form or food (e.g. bananas, sports bars, carbohydrate gels) or sports drinks (e.g. Gatorade™, PowerAde™). If carbohydrate is consumed then the reliance on slowly digesting carbohydrate from the low GI meal is not as important as blood glucose levels will be maintained by the high carbohydrate foods (usually of a high GI, see page 55) that are consumed regularly during exercise. As most endurance athletes would do this and event organisers provide aid stations to support refuelling along the course, the application of the low GI pre-event meal may not be as wide as first thought.

Some athletes however may still benefit from a low GI pre-event meal if they have abnormal glucose tolerance or in particular a tendency to experience low blood glucose especially after eating meals with a high GI. This condition is known as hypoglycaemia. It is definitely worth these athletes experimenting with low GI meals prior to exercise. Before the event, these athletes should choose low GI foods that are not too fibrous or 'gas producing'—taking a 'pit stop' at the loo during exercise can be very inconvenient. Suitable light and low GI foods include pasta, some varieties of rice (Basmati, Doongara), low GI breads (those with barley or wholegrains) and some breakfast cereals (e.g. porridge).

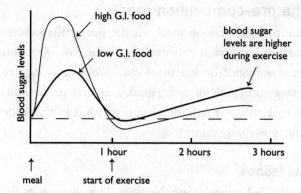

Figure 4: Comparison of the effect of low and high GI foods on blood sugar levels during prolonged strenuous exercise. When a pre-event meal of lentils (low GI) was compared with potatoes (high GI), cyclists were able to continue cycling at a high intensity (65 per cent of their peak aerobic capacity) for 20 minutes longer after eating the lentil meal. Their blood sugar and insulin levels were significantly higher at the end of exercise, indicating that carbohydrate was still being absorbed from the small intestine ever after 90 minutes of strenuous exercise.

The pre-competition meal

The pre-competition meal has the potential to either make or break your performance on the day. What you eat should not be left to chance. Work on a dietary strategy using the following guidelines, then practise this strategy before a training session so you can fine tune your pre-competition meal.

Guidelines

- Eat 2–4 hours before the event. This allows time for your pre-competition meal to be emptied from the stomach. Allow 4 hours for a larger meal.
- Make the meal high in carbohydrate for maximum energy.
- Top up, do not over eat. Eat a comfortable amount of food.
- Keep the fat down in this meal. Fat slows digestion.
- Moderate protein, fill up on carbohydrates instead.
- Moderate fibre, too much high fibre food could cause bloating, diarrhoea and discomfort during competition. Leave your high-fibre eating for non-competition days.
- Drink your meal, if you're nervous, or you feel it's too early in the morning to eat, try a sports drink or liquid meal type drink (e.g. Sustagen™) so that you can maintain your energy with liquid food.

• Practise, experiment with different meals to find out what works best for you.

On your mark

Remember, the pre-event meal won't work miracles if your training diet is inadequate. Make sure you are eating well generally, especially for the week leading up to competition.

Get set

Use these pre-competition guidelines to help you plan your pre-event meal.

Go

During exercise, replace fluids and carbohydrates regularly as you go.

DURING THE EVENT

High GI carbohydrate is the best choice to optimise performance as the carbohydrate needs to be rapidly available to the muscle as a fuel source. Consuming carbohydrate 'on the run' has been shown to delay fatigue as it provides energy to working muscles when the body's own stores of glycogen are low. This is especially the case when exercise is prolonged and even glycogen loading cannot prepare the body for the carbohydrate needed to get through the long endurance event.

Prolong your endurance
by topping up fluids and carbohydrate
regularly throughout exercise.

If you don't have sufficient carbohydrate in your training diet, supplementing carbohydrate during exercise helps you keep pace when your glycogen stores are low. This is not a quick fix to avoid a high carbohydrate training diet! The body prefers to obtain carbs from glycogen stored in the muscle during exercise. Outside carbs are a great back up, but it's still essential to prepare your body by eating a high carb training diet each day.

The table below lists high GI carbohydrates that are popular during exercise. Sports electrolyte replacement drinks are a great choice as they are emptied quickly from the stomach and also aid hydration as well.

During exercise: high GI choices

Food	GI	Serving size	Carbohydrate (g)
Sport drink (electrolyte)	73–78	1 litre	60–80
White bread with honey	70	2 slices with 2 tsp honey	40
Breakfast bar (fruit flavour)	78	1 bar	29
Jelly beans	80	100 g	60
Rice cakes	82	5 cakes	50
Scones	70	2 large	50

Sports or electrolyte replacement drinks are ideal as they encourage greater fluid consumption than water, enhance intestinal absorption of fluid and provide carbohydrate while rehydrating the body at the same time.

Sports drinks

	GI	Nominal Serve Size	Available Carb Per Serve	GL
Gatorade®	78	250 ml	15	12
Powerade®	65	250 ml	20	13

The choice of solid or liquid carbohydrate during exercise is ultimately up to the individual, however, with the current sports/electrolyte formulations providing an optimal quickly absorbed source of carbs, it is hard to look past this as a primary option. Many exercisers choose a combination of sports drinks and comfortable solid foods they have trialled in training. Solids help in prolonged exercise to fill that 'empty' feeling in the stomach.

Many of the popular foods used during exercise over the years were adopted because they were convenient or easy to eat, rather than because they had a high GI. The ever popular banana for example has an intermediate GI. Eating a banana during exercise is not wrong. However, when the pace is really on and you want a fast energy supply, a faster absorbing high GI option would technically be better. In prolonged exercise, you should aim to consume 30–60 grams of carbohydrate per hour over the session (or event).

In long events, a combination of comfortable foods whatever their GI along with the high GI options will provide the best variety and feelings of psychological well being. The occasional mini chocolate bar as a treat may not scientifically be the best, highest GI fuel during exercise, but in the final stages of the ironman, it may boost your morale enough to keep you going. These psychological factors cannot be underestimated.

AFTER THE EVENT: RECOVERY

After exercise, your muscles are hungry for carbohydrate. Postponing carbohydrate consumption after exercise delays muscle glycogen replenishment and can cause fatigue.

In the immediate post-exercise period, high GI carbohydrates are best because they are digested and absorbed much faster and stimulate more insulin—the hormone responsible for getting glucose into the muscle and storing it as glycogen. Most athletes prefer high carbohydrate drinks because they are usually thirsty rather than hungry after strenuous exercise. A drink also aids rehydration.

Sports or electrolyte replacement drinks are ideal for replacing fluids and providing an immediate and convenient source of high GI carbohydrate.

After this initial 'hit' of recovery carbs, try to make sure your next meal or snack (within 2 hours) includes intermediate to high GI foods.

- If you are a recreational exerciser, an adequate carbohydrate intake over the next few days will ensure that muscles are ready for another session.

- If you are participating in strenuous training, particularly when two or more training sessions are part of the daily routine, rapid glycogen replenishment is vital. Eat or drink carbohydrate (within 30 minutes) after strenuous exercise when another training session is on the agenda a few hours later. On consecutive days of competition, this recovery strategy will also assist in restocking your glycogen stores for the next event.

Recovery formula

The amount of carbohydrate required to kick off the recovery process in the first two hours is about 1 gram per kilogram of body weight. Most people need between 50 to 100 grams of carbohydrate in the immediate post-exercise period. The following table outlines a list of convenient high GI foods and sports drinks, suitable for recovery.

> Postponing carbohydrate consumption
> after exercise delays muscle glycogen
> replenishment and can cause fatigue.

Females weighing about 50 kilograms should aim to eat 50 grams of carbohydrate.

Males weighing about 75 kilograms should aim to eat 75 grams of carbohydrate.

High GI foods to enhance recovery

Food	GI	Serving size = 50 grams carbohydrate	Serving size = 75 grams carbohydrate
White or brown bread	70	100 g (3 slices)	150 g (4–5 slices)
Rice bubbles (Kelloggs®)	89	45 g (1½ cups + 175 ml milk)	65 g (2 cups + 300 ml milk)
Cornflakes (Kelloggs®)	84	45 g (1½ cups + 175 ml milk)	65 g (2 cups + 300 ml milk)
Scones	70	150 g (2 large scones)	200 g (3 large scones)
Morning coffee biscuits	79	65 g (10 biscuits)	100 g (15 biscuits)
Rice cakes	82	60 g (5 rice cakes)	90 g (8 rice cakes)
Muffins (English-style, toasted)	70	120 g (2 muffins)	180 g (3 muffins)
Rice (Calrose), cooked	83	180 g (1 cup)	270 g (1½ cups)
Jelly beans	80	54 g (6 jelly beans)	81 g (9 jelly beans)
Sports electrolyte drink 6% carb	73–78	850 ml	1250 ml

CASE STUDY 1: NATHAN

Nathan is an 18-year-old Australian Rules football player. He recently moved from a small country town to take up a position in one of the best sides in the league. Playing professional footy was Nathan's dream. Wanting to make a big impression during his first few weeks at training, Nathan gave his all. At first he felt fine, but after one week of training twice almost every day he felt exhausted, and was frankly 'off the pace'. Sensing that Nathan was struggling, the coach took him aside and recommended he speak to the club's sports dietitian about his diet and recovery strategies.

Nathan's Weekly Training Program

Morning weight/circuit training;
2–3 sessions per week of 1–1.5 hours

Afternoon football/fitness sessions:
4 sessions of 2–2.5 hours per week

Consultation with the sports dietitian

Nathan was as bit wary, he wondered what diet could really do for him. The dietitian explained that carbohydrates were the key to energy and recovery. His diet at the moment was far too low in carbohydrate to get him through the tough pre-season training. The dietitian also explained that eating carbohydrate regularly was important, and fuelling up immediately (within 30 minutes) after training sessions helped to replace the body's carbohydrate stores more quickly. Timing was important because between morning and afternoon training his body had less than 6 hours to refuel. More rapidly absorbing carbs or those with an intermediate to high GI were also better for refuelling as they replenished the body's carbohydrate or glycogen levels faster.

The dietitian also explained that to help Nathan maintain his body weight and stay lean he should:

• use lean meats or cut off the fat
• remove chicken skin from chicken
• use reduced fat dairy products
• minimise use of oils, butter or margarine

High GI fuel to the rescue

Nathan noticed the other players in his team were already consuming sports drinks with glucose (high GI) to begin the refuelling and rehydration process straight after training and chose intermediate to high GI breads, cereals or fruit to boost their recovery (French bread, Weet-Bix™, Wheatbites™, Breakfast Bar™, pineapple, watermelon). These foods were available at training so he could start the refuelling process before travelling home.

The dietitian also organised cooking classes to give him confidence preparing different carbohydrate-based meals for himself. But Nathan now knew that when recovery time was short, higher carbohydrates were best.

Results

Nathan noticed the difference in his performance after being on the high carbohydrate diet for only a few days. He felt fresher at afternoon training and could really power through the sprint sessions which had been like torture before. Including more carbohydrate in his diet and refuelling with higher GI carbohydrates really helped him. He knew he still had a lot of work to do before the competition season kicked off but with the right fuel, a great attitude and some raw talent he reckoned he was ready for some of his best ever performances.

Meal plan for Nathan

Aim: To provide sufficient carbohydrate and energy and to assist recovery rate by incorporating high GI liquids and intermediate-to-high GI meals after training.

8.30 am	Immediately post-training
1 litre sports/electrolyte drink	

9.00 am   Breakfast:

1 piece fruit

2 cups of cereal

2 cups of reduced fat milk

2 slices white or wholemeal toast (no butter) with honey

1 glass of fruit juice

Post-training Intermediate-to-high GI choices

Pineapple, Watermelon

Puffed wheat, Weet-bix, Wheatbites

White or wholemeal with a high GI (see tables)

French bread has a high GI

Pineapple is his favourite juice

11.30 am   Snack

1 sandwich (no butter) lean meat filling

1 piece of fruit (any type)

low fat yoghurt

1.00 pm   Lunch
3 salad sandwiches or rolls filled
with any of the following: lean meat,
chicken, reduced fat cheese, egg,
canned tuna in spring water or
canned salmon
2 pieces of fresh fruit (any type)
600 ml of reduced fat, flavoured
milk

2.30 pm   *Snack*
Fruit smoothie or a liquid meal
(e.g. Sustagen™)

4.30–5.30 pm   **Pre- and during   High GI (73–78)
                     training**
2–3 litres of sports/electrolyte drink

5.30 pm   **After training: High GI for recovery
1 litre sports/electrolyte drink or
carb loader

7.00 pm.   Dinner

Large serving lean meat (155 g), or
skinless chicken (185 g), or fish
(250 g) grilled or cooked with
minimum oil

Large serving of rice, or pasta or potato	High GI rice on training nights, pasta most others
Medium serving of vegetable or tossed green salad (no-oil dressing)	
4 slices of white bread or 2 rolls (no butter)	High GI French bread on training nights

9.00 pm   *Snack*

2 pieces of fresh fruit in a smoothie
or fruit and yoghurt

Dietary analysis

Energy:	18 821 kilojoules (4480 calories)
Protein:	194 g (17 per cent)
Fat:	67 g (14 per cent)
Carbohydrate:	775 g (69 per cent)

CASE STUDY 2: IAN

Ian is a 26-year-old physical education teacher and keen triathlete. He has competed in the Olympic distance for the past 5 years but is now keen to qualify for the ironman triathlon in Hawaii. Ian wanted everything to be spot on for his first ironman race so he could qualify for Hawaii. He approached a sports dietitian to help him plan his dietary strategy and brought a list of questions to ask.

Ian's Vital Statistics

Height 178 cm

Weight 75 kg (has lost 4 kg over the past 3 months)

Sum of 8 skinfolds 50 mm (indicates that Ian is very lean)

How much carbohydrate does he need in his training diet?

The approximate amount of carbohydrate Ian needs is calculated by multiplying his weight by the carbohydrate requirement appropriate for his activity level.

Ian's weight   75 kg
Approximate carbohydrate
    requirement for his activity level
    (see page 27–8)   8 g/kg
Daily carbohydrate needs for
    training   75 × 8 = 600 g

This amount of carbohydrate may be too difficult to achieve with food. Liquid carbohydrate supplements like sports drinks can help boost carbohydrate intake.

Ian's training program

	AM TRAINING	PM TRAINING
Monday	3 km swim	Track session + 15 km run
Tuesday	3 km swim	100 km cycle
Wednesday	Rest	15 km run
Thursday	3 km swim	100 km cycle
Friday	3 km swim	50 km easy cycle
Saturday	150 km cycle	3 km swim
Sunday	Rest	30 km run

How can he incorporate the GI into his training diet?

Ian can incorporate the GI into his diet mainly by including high GI drinks (e.g. sports drinks) during and after training. Intermediate-to-high GI foods after training also help to speed up recovery. At other times, the most important thing is to eat sufficient carbohydrate, whatever the GI. (Most athletes requiring the amount of carbohydrate that Ian does will feel more comfortable with moderate-to-lower fibre carbohydrate choices (e.g. white bread, white rice and pasta instead of the wholegrain varieties). Otherwise the sheer volume of the carbohydrate and fibre becomes too bulky and bloating.

Why was he so fatigued lately?

Fatigue is a generalised symptom that has numerous causes. Dietary facts that should be considered include:

- Low iron intake. If this is low, then increased amounts of high iron foods need to be included in the diet. Iron deficiency even in athletes with adequate iron intake does occur, and is more common in endurance athletes.

- Inadequate carbohydrate intake. Fatigue can be experienced if muscle glycogen stores are low indicating inadequate intake of carbohydrate over the day. Tiredness can also be due to low blood glucose. This may occur if there is a long period between meals. Low blood glucose (hypoglycaemia) commonly occurs in early morning or afternoon training sessions where insufficient carbohydrate is consumed before the session.

- Overtraining is a common problem with endurance athletes. Training programs need to be tailored to the individual, incorporating their personal needs for sleep and taking into account their occupational demands.

Viral illness and a number of other medical conditions are also potential causes of fatigue. Ian would benefit from a referral to a sports physician and an exercise scientist to investigate which factors in particular are causing his fatigue.

Does he need to glycogen load prior to the event?

Since the event will be longer than 2 hours (about 11 hours actually), yes! The meal plan outlines how he can glycogen load using the modified regimen. This regimen involves tapered training and a high carbohydrate diet 3–4 days prior to the race. The diet should provide about 9–10 g of carbohydrate per kg of body weight. Check the meal plan for guidance.

What would be the best pre-event meal?

Ian could try a low GI meal in practice to see how this worked for him although as he plans to use sports drinks and high GI foods during the event it may not be necessary. To maintain gastric comfort, the best low GI options would include lower fibre choices such as, white pasta, rolled oats, or a liquid low fat milk based meal (Sustagen Sport™).

How could he maintain energy throughout the event?

During the event, maintaining energy and hydration will be a major factor influencing his performance. Sports drinks would be the best option to replace energy and fluids during the race. As sports drinks have a high GI, they will be a rapidly absorbed and easily available source of carbohydrate. Other high GI options include carbohydrate gels, jelly beans, honey sandwiches on high GI (white) bread. As Ian will only be able to carry a small amount of the high GI food options, the sports drink will probably provide the basis of his refuelling strategy with foods offering minor support.

To prevent boredom and as a morale booster some of the other offerings at the aid stations (choc chip cookies, jam sandwich, cola drink) could be included in smaller quantities as treats. These provide more of a psychological incentive than physiological boost. Although a little caffeine in the cola drink may help with fatigue later in the race due to its stimulant properties. Ian needs to limit caffeine ingestion to avoid problems with its dehydration effect and slower stomach emptying which may compromise hydration. Caffeine is also subject to drug testing.

Ian's meal plan

Aim: To provide sufficient carbohydrate and nutrition for peak performance. The meal plan should include intermediate to high GI meals or snacks after training sessions to help maximise the rate of glycogen replacement.

Regular training	Notes on GI	Loading phase
	Intermediate-to-high GI post-training	

Breakfast

1–2 pieces of fresh fruit	Pineapple, watermelon Weet-bix, Puffed Wheat, Wheatbites	Same breakfast
2 cups cereal		
1 cup reduced fat milk	High GI bread (e.g. regular white bread)	
3 slices of toast with honey (no butter)	Pineapple	
500 ml fruit juice		

Snack

1 banana and honey roll	As for training plan but add in an additional banana roll or a healthy fruit muffin
1 glass (250 ml) juice (any type)	

Regular training	*Notes on GI* *Intermediate-to-high* *GI Post-training*	*Loading phase*

Lunch

3 sandwiches with
salad (including cheese,
chicken, lean meat, egg,
tuna or salmon as
for fillings)
1 piece fruit
1 glass sports drink

Same lunch but
add in a honey
or jam sandwich
for extra
carbohydrate

Snack

As for morning tea or
a fruit smoothie
Before and during
training
Sports drink (volume
dependent on session
type and duration)

Use a liquid meal
e.g., Sustagen™
or carb loader.
Ensure adequate
fluid replacement

Regular training	Notes on GI Intermediate-to-high GI Post-training	Loading phase
Dinner		
Medium serving of lean meat (125 g), skinless chicken (155 g), fish (200 g) or a vegetarian meal Large serving of potato, rice or pasta Medium serving of vegetable or tossed green salad, no-oil dressing. 4 slices of bread or two rolls 2 pieces of fresh fruit 1 glass (250 ml) juice (any)	High GI rice, great after hard afternoon training sessions, High GI bread Pineapple, watermelon	Same dinner
Supper		
4 pieces raisin toast with jam or honey 1 glass fruit juice		Add in a carb-loader drink or a liquid meal e.g., Sustagen™

Dietary analysis (training)	Dietary analysis (loading)
Energy: 16 700 kilojoules (3977 calories)	**Energy:** 18 925 kilojoules (4500 calories)
Protein: 179 g (18 per cent)	**Protein:** 195 g (17 per cent)
Fat: 85 g (19 per cent)	**Fat:** 85 g (16 per cent)
Carbohydrate: 624 g (63 per cent)	**Carbohydrate:** 745 g (67 per cent)

The pre-event meal plan for Ian

This meal should be consumed about 2–3 hours prior to competition. Ian had tried out the low GI meal in training and wanted to use it in competition. The meals he found most comfortable included:

- Liquid meal (Sustagen Sport™)
  plus a serving of stewed apple   GI = 39
- Rolled oats with skim milk and
  orange juice   GI = 44
- Tinned spaghetti on grain
  bread toast   GI = 47

Results

Ian went on to qualify for Hawaii. Being prepared for this race was crucial to best performance. The Hawaii Ironman was 'awesome'—one of his best-ever life-experiences that was made more enjoyable by being well-prepared and well-fuelled.

WEIGHT CONTROL EATING

Athletes train hard so it comes as a surprise to find that many of them need to watch their weight or body fat levels. This is often because in some sports the level of weight or leanness required is extreme. Gymnasts, ballet dancers, triathletes and endurance runners need to be light and lean to participate in their sport at the elite level. In other sports (e.g. jockeys, boxers, martial arts and light weight rowing) athletes may need to make a weight to compete. Sometimes being extremely lean is purely for aesthetic purposes (e.g. body building).

Some athletes find it harder than others to achieve the right weight and body fat level for their sport. A diet with a low GI may help these athletes as it can help them to stay fuller and more satisfied, making it easier not to overconsume foods, particularly those high in fat.

In the past, it was believed that protein, fat and carbohydrate foods, taken in equal quantities, satisfy our appetite equally. We now know from recent research that the satiating capacity—the degree to which foods make us feel full—of these nutrients is not equal.

Fatty food, in particular, has only a weak effect on satisfying appetite relative to the number of kilojoules they provide. This has been demonstrated clearly in experimental situations where people are asked to eat until their appetite is satisfied. They over-consume kilojoules if the foods they are offered are high in fat. When high carbohydrate and low fat foods are offered, they consume few kilojoules when given the opportunity to eat until satisfied. So, carbohydrate foods are the best for satisfying your appetite without over-satisfying your kilojoule requirement.

Low GI foods fill you up and keep you satisfied for longer

In studies we conducted, people were given a range of individual foods that contained equal numbers of kilojoules, then their satiety responses were compared. We found that the most filling foods were those that contained fewer kilojoules per gram, in other words, the least energy dense. This included potatoes, porridge, apples, oranges and pasta. Eating more of these foods satisfies appetite without providing excess kilojoules. On the other hand, foods that provide a lot of kilojoules per gram, like croissants, chocolate and peanuts, were the least satisfying. These foods are more likely to leave us wanting more and to lead to what scientist call 'passive overconsumption', i.e. overeating without realising it.

After energy density, the second best predictor of satiety was a food's GI—the lower the GI, the more the food satisfied people's hunger. Indeed, there are now over 17 studies that confirm low GI foods are able to suppress hunger for longer than high GI foods.

There are probably several mechanisms responsible for this.

- Low GI foods remain longer in the small intestine, triggering receptors that tell the brain there's food still in the gut to be digested.
- High GI foods may stimulate hunger because the rapid rise and then fall in blood glucose levels appears to stimulate counter-regulatory responses to reverse the decline.
- Stress hormones like adrenalin and cortisol are released when glucose levels rebound after a high GI food. Both hormones tend to stimulate appetite.
- Low GI foods may be more satiating simply because they are often less energy dense than their high GI counterparts. The naturally high fibre content of

many low GI foods increases their bulk without increasing their energy content.

What's more, even when the kilojoule intake is the same, people eating low GI foods may lose more weight than those eating high GI foods. In a South African study, the investigators divided overweight volunteers into two groups: one group ate high GI foods and the other, low GI foods. The amount of kilojoules, fat, protein, carbohydrate and fibre in the diet was the same for both groups. Only the GI of the diets was different. The low GI group included foods like lentils, pasta, porridge and corn in their diet and excluded high GI foods like potato and white bread. After 12 weeks, the volunteers in the group eating low GI foods had lost, on average, 9 kilograms—2 kilograms more than people in the group eating the diet of high GI foods.

How did the low GI diet work? The most significant finding was the different effects of the two diets on the level of insulin in the blood. Low GI foods resulted in lower levels of insulin circulating in the bloodstream. Insulin is a hormone that is not only involved in regulating blood sugar levels, it also plays a key part in when and how we store fat. High levels of insulin often exist in obese people, in those with high blood fat levels (either cholesterol or triglyceride) and those with heart disease. This study suggested that the low insulin responses associated with low GI foods helped the body to burn more fat rather than store it.

There are other reasons why low GI diets might aid weight loss. When people first begin a diet, their metabolic rate drops in response to the reduction in food intake. One study, however, found that the metabolic rate had dropped less after one week on a low GI diet compared to a conventional high carbohydrate diet. The same study suggested that the low GI diet helped to preserve lean body mass better, which could explain the higher metabolic rate.

CASE STUDY 3: ANALISE

Analise, a 16-year-old full-time ballet student, had a dream: to be a dancer with the Australian Ballet Company. When she started to mature at 13, she found she could no longer 'eat anything'. Extra weight started to pile on. First she tried all the diets given to her by the other ballet students. Getting nowhere fast by herself, her mother took her to see a sports dietitian.

Consultation with the sports dietitian

At their first meeting the dietitian took a history of Analise's weight and eating patterns and found that a typical day's meals included:

1 slice of white toast with butter and a cup of strong black tea for breakfast

2 crispbreads with butter and a cup of black tea for a morning snack

1 green salad, an apple and a cup of black tea for lunch

1 chocolate bar and a can of diet cola during the afternoon (waiting at the train station)

Steamed veges, sometimes steamed chicken and a cup of black tea for dinner

1 chocolate bar or chocolate biscuits and tea for supper.

The dietitian explained that this diet was high in fat and too low in protein, carbohydrate, calcium and iron. She explained that:

- Gaining a little body weight and fat is part of the maturation process and that the best way to control body fat was with a sensible diet, not starving.

- Cravings are to be expected when you are hungry. After working hard in class all day with virtually no food, chocolate is just too tempting. Eating more carbohydrate on a regular basis would help Analise control her chocolate cravings.

- Analise needed a dietary strategy to give her sufficient fuel to get through the day without feeling hungry. Carbohydrates (especially crunchy and chewy carbs with a low GI) would help her to feel fuller (satiety), give her more energy and are much less fattening than fats.

Analise's meal plan, based on reducing fat intake and boosting carbohydrate, meant eating more pasta, rice, bread, fruit and vegetables and less high fat food like butter and chocolate. Chocolate was not totally out but she had to cut back to get her body fat levels going in the right direction. The dietitian also explained that drinking less tea would help Analise maintain adequate iron levels. The tannin in tea reduces iron absorption.

Analise had some questions about the meal plan.

Could she really lose weight eating this much?
The dietitian explained that the size or appearance of foods is often deceiving. Although some high fat foods like chocolate look compact, and foods like bread and vegetables may take up more space on the plate, the fat and kilojoule (calorie) value of high fat foods is much more than bread and vegetables. The fat figures in the back of this book were a real surprise to Analise as was the fact that the fat we eat is converted into body fat, faster and easier than anything else we eat.

Should she cut out chocolate all together?
The dietitian explained that giving up chocolate is really not necessary and is almost impossible unless you live somewhere where there's no chocolate at all. Eating chocolate as a treat rather than a substitute meal is the key.

How could she avoid feeling too full and having a bloated stomach during class?

Foods with a high fibre content (including many salad veges) may produce more gas in the intestine and this can cause bloating. The dietitian showed how Analise could increase the intake of low GI carbs through the day without bloating.

Results

At first Analise kept thinking that she was eating too much. But she found avoiding the chocolate vending machine on the station platform on the way home easier because she felt fuller through the day as the high carb, low GI foods reduced her hunger. Her body fat level (measured with body fat or skinfold callipers) dropped steadily each fortnight. It was almost unbelievable to be able to drop fat without starving. An added bonus was her improved energy levels and concentration in class, not to mention her mood which was more relaxed and cheerful.

Analise's meal plan

Aim: To provide a regular supply of carbohydrate, with less fat. The GI to be intermediate to low to assist with satiety.

8.00 am **Breakfast**	**Intermediate to low GI**
1 piece of fruit	Fresh apple, grapefruit,
1 cup bran cereal	kiwi fruit
1 slice wholegrain	All Bran, oats, Sultana Bran™
toast (no butter) and jam	Oat, barley, mixed
1 cup decaffeinated coffee	grain or fruit breads

10.30 am *Snack*	
1 piece of fruit or a low	Fruit like, apricot, cherries,
fat fruit yoghurt	orange

1.00 pm **Lunch**	
1 sandwich (no butter).	Oat, barley or heavy
Protein options include:,	grain bread
chicken, turkey, canned tuna	
in brine or water, salmon,	
reduced fat cheese, lean ham,	
corn beef or roast meat.	
Small amount of salad	Peach, pear or plum
1 piece of fruit	
Water or a low joule drink	
(not containing caffeine)	

3.30 pm   *Snack*

1 raisin toast with jam or   Raisin bread or grain
½ English muffin with jam.   muffin
Or fruit or low fat yoghurt
as in morning snack

7.00 pm   Dinner

Small serving of lean meat   New boiled potatoes,
(90 g), or skinless chicken   pasta, Basmati or
(125 g) or grilled fish (155 g).   Doongara rice
All cooked in minimum to no
oil. 2 potatoes or pasta
or Basmati or Doongara rice
Large serving of vegetables or
salad with low oil dressing
Water or low joule cordial

9.30 pm   Supper

1 glass of reduced fat milk
1 slice of raisin toast with jam

Dietary analysis

Energy:	5640 kilojoules (1300 calories)
Protein:	80 g (24 per cent)
Fat:	20 g (14 per cent)
Carbohydrate:	208 g (62 per cent)
Calcium:	800 mg (equal to the recommended daily intake)
Iron:	14–18 mg (above the recommended daily intake)

YOUR QUESTIONS ANSWERED

What should be the overall GI of an athlete's diet?
This is a good question and one the scientists are yet to answer. There is evidence that diets with a higher GI increase the glycogen storage in the muscle of sedentary individuals. This may help athletes to store glycogen more effectively on a day to day basis. A high GI has been shown to enhance the rate of recovery of muscle glycogen after exercise. During exercise, a high GI is required to provide a rapidly available fuel source.

I am a recreational jogger, what should be the GI of my overall diet?
If the exercise is undertaken as part of a weight loss program, there may be some benefit in choosing low GI carbohydrates at each meal for their higher satiety

value. In general for recreational joggers, it is important to have sufficient carbohydrate in the diet for good health and energy. Since the time to restore glycogen after a work out is likely to be longer than for elite athletes, there is less need to have high GI carbohydrates immediately after exercise.

What about the pre-event meal before high intensity or non-endurance exercise?

As mentioned there is evidence that low GI carbohydrates before endurance exercise may help to enhance performance. Studies on shorter term exercise have not been done so we need to await further research. At this stage, there are many factors to consider in planning an optimal pre-event meal. The timing, the fibre content so as to prevent bloating, the fat content and of course the GI. Much of the advice about pre-event eating has come from practical experience, and surprisingly little from scientific research. As so many factors need to be considered, the best advice for shorter term exercise at present is for individuals to consider the list of optimal pre-event eating strategies and experiment with foods or meals to determine what works best for them.

What about eating between heats and trials over the day?

It makes sense to include carbohydrates that are rapidly absorbed (i.e. higher GI) on a regular basis over the day. Eat little and often. Maintain fluid intake to optimise hydration. In shorter breaks, rapidly absorbed liquids are probably best. In longer breaks (more than 1 hour), small, low fat, high carb snacks (e.g. rice cakes, soft fruits, honey sandwiches, sports bars etc.) are recommended.

LET'S TALK GLYCEMIC LOAD

When we eat a meal containing carbohydrate, the blood glucose rises and falls. The extent to which it rises and remains high is critically important to health and depends on two things: the amount of a carbohydrate in the meal and the nature (GI) of that carbohydrate. Both are equally important determinants of changes in blood glucose levels.

Researchers at Harvard University came up with a way of combining and describing these two factors with the term 'glycemic load'. Glycemic load (GL) is the product of the GI and carbohydrate per serve of food. You'll find it in the tables at the back of this book.

Glycemic load is calculated simply by multiplying the GI of a food by the amount of carbohydrate per serving and dividing by 100.

Glycemic load = (GI x carbohydrate per
serving) ÷ 100

For example, an apple has a GI of 40 and contains
15 grams of carbohydrate per serve. Its glycemic load is
$(40 \times 15) \div 100 = 6$. A potato has a GI of 90 and 20
grams of carbohydrate per serve. It has a glycemic load
of $(90 \times 20) \div 100 = 18$.

The glycemic load is greatest for those foods which
provide the most carbohydrate, particularly those we
tend to eat in large quantities. Compare the glycemic
load of the following foods to see how the serving size
as well as the GI are significant in determining the
glycemic response:

- Rice—1 cup of boiled Calrose rice (150 g) contains
  43 g carbohydrate and has a GI of 83. The glycemic
  load is $(83 \times 43) \div 100 = 36$.
- Spaghetti—1 serve (150 g) of cooked spaghetti
  contains 48 g carbohydrate and has a GI of 44. The
  glycemic load is $(44 \times 48) \div 100 = 21$.

Some nutritionists have argued that the glycemic
load is an improvement on the GI because it provides
an estimate of both quantity and quality of carbohydrate
(the GI gives us just quality) in a diet. In large scale
studies from Harvard University, however, the risk of
disease was predicted by both the GI of the overall diet

as well as the glycemic load. The use of the glycemic load strengthened the relationship, suggesting that the more frequent the consumption of high carbohydrate, high GI foods, the more adverse the health outcome.

Don't make the mistake of using GL alone. If you do, you might find yourself eating a diet with very little carbohydrate but a lot of fat, especially staurated fat, and excessive amounts of protein. Use the glycemic index to compare foods of similar nature (e.g. bread with bread) and use the glycemic load when you note a high GI but low carbohydrate content per serve (e.g. pumpkin).

THE GI & GL TABLES

These tables are an A to Z listing of the GI and GL of foods commonly eaten in Australia and New Zealand. Approximately 400 different foods are listed.

The GI value shown next to each food is the average for that food using glucose as the standard, i.e., glucose has a GI value of 100, with other foods rated accordingly. The average may represent the mean of ten studies of that food worldwide or only two to four studies. In a few instances, Australian data are different from the rest of the world and we show our data rather than the average. Rice and porridge fall into this category.

The glycemic load (GL = carbohydrate content × GI ÷ 100) shows you the blood glucose response to a serving of a food. The higher the glycemic load the higher your blood glucose level will rise. This is calculated using a 'nominal' serving size and the carbohydrate content of that serve, both of which are also listed in the tables. In this way, you can choose foods with either a low GI and/or a low GL.

We've also included foods that contain very little carbohydrate and have therefore been automatically omitted from previous editions. However, so many people ask us for the GI of these foods, we decided to include them and show their GI as 0, indicated by a zero [0]. Many vegetables such as avocados and broccoli and protein foods such as chicken, cheese and tuna are among the low or no carbohydrate category.

If you can't find a GI value for a food you eat regularly, please write to the manufacturer and encourage them to have the GI of the food tested by an accredited laboratory such as Sydney University Glycemic Index Research Service (SUGiRS) (www.glycemicindex.com).

You might also encourage companies to join the GI symbol program (www.gisymbol.com.au), which flags healthy foods that have been properly tested.

The GI values in these tables are correct at the time of publication. However, the formulation of commercial foods can change and the GI may be altered. You can rely on those foods showing the GI symbol. You will find revised and new data on our webpage (www.glycemicindex.com).

FOOD	GI	NOMINAL SERVE SIZE	AVAILABLE CARB PER SERVE	GL PER SERVE
All-Bran™, breakfast cereal	30	30 g	15	4
All-Bran Fruit 'n' Oats™, breakfast cereal	39	30 g	17	7
All-Bran Soy 'n' Fibre™, breakfast cereal	33	30 g	14	4
Angel food cake, 1 slice	67	50 g	29	19
Apple, raw, 1 medium	38*	120 g	15	6
Apple, dried	29	60 g	34	10
Apple juice, pure, unsweetened	40	250 ml	28	11
Apple muffin	44	60 g	29	13
Apple, oat and sultana muffin (from packet mix)	54	50 g	26	14
Apricots, raw, 3 medium	57	168 g	13	7
Apricots, canned in light syrup	64	120 g	19	12
Apricots, dried	30	60 g	27	8
Apricot, coconut and honey muffin (from mix)	60	50 g	26	16
Arborio, risotto rice, white, boiled	69	150 g	43	29
Bagel, white	72	70 g	35	25
Baked beans, canned in tomato sauce	48*	150 g	17	8
Banana, raw, 1 large	52*	120 g	26	13
Banana cake, 1 slice	47	80 g	38	18
Banana, oat and honey muffin (from packet mix)	65	50 g	26	17
Barley, pearled, boiled	25*	150 g	32	8
Basmati rice, white, boiled, 1 cup	58	150 g	42	24
Beef	[0]	120 g	0	0
Beer	[0]	150 ml	0	0

* Average

FOOD	GI	NOMINAL SERVE SIZE	AVAILABLE CARB PER SERVE	GL PER SERVE
Beetroot, canned	64	80 g	7	5
Bengal gram dhal, chickpea	11	150 g	36	4
Black bean soup	64	250 ml	27	17
Black beans, boiled	30	150 g	25	5
Blackbread (Riga)	76	30 g	13	10
Blackeyed beans, soaked, boiled	42	150 g	29	12
Blueberry muffin	59	57 g	29	17
Bran Flakes™, breakfast cereal	74	30 g	18	13
Bran muffin	60	57 g	24	15
Breton™ wheat crackers	67	25 g	14	10
Broad beans	79	80 g	11	9
Broken rice, white, cooked in rice cooker	86	150 g	43	37
Buckwheat, boiled	54*	150 g	30	16
Buckwheat, pancakes, gluten-free, made from packet mix	102	77 g	22	22
Bulghur, boiled 20 min	48*	150 g	26	12
Bun, hamburger	61	30 g	15	9
Bürgen® Oat Bran & Honey	49	40 g	13	7
Bürgen® Soy-Lin, kibbled soy (8%) and linseed (8%) loaf	36	30 g	9	3
Bürgen® Fruit Loaf	44	30 g	13	6
Bürgen® Mixed Grain	49*	30 g	11	6
Burger Rings™, barbeque-flavoured	90	50 g	31	28
Butter beans, dried, boiled	31*	150 g	20	6
Calrose rice, white, medium grain, boiled	83	150 g	42	35
Capellini pasta, boiled	45	180 g	45	20

* Average

FOOD	GI	NOMINAL SERVE SIZE	AVAILABLE CARB PER SERVE	GL PER SERVE
Capsicum	[0]	80 g	0	0
Carrots, peeled, boiled	41*	80 g	5	2
Cheese	[0]	120 g	0	0
Cherries, raw	63	60 g	6	4
Chickpeas, canned in brine	42	150 g	22	9
Chickpeas, dried, boiled	28*	150 g	24	7
Chicken nuggets, frozen, reheated in microwave oven 5 min	46	100 g	16	7
Chocolate, plain, milk	43*	50 g	28	12
Chocolate, white, Milky Bar®	44	50 g	29	13
Chocolate butterscotch muffins, made from packet mix	53	50 g	28	15
Chocolate cake made from packet mix with chocolate frosting	38	111 g	52	20
Chocolate mousse, 2% fat	31	50 g	11	3
Chocolate pudding, instant made from packet with whole milk	47	100 g	16	7
Coca Cola®, soft drink	53	250 ml	26	14
Coco Pops™	77	30 g	26	20
Condensed milk, sweetened, full-fat	61	50 ml	28	17
Cordial, orange, reconstituted	66	250 ml	20	13
Corn chips, plain, salted	42	50 g	25	11
Cornflakes™, breakfast cereal	77	30 g	25	20
Cornflakes Crunchy Nut™, breakfast cereal	72	30 g	24	17
Cornmeal, boiled in salted water 2 min	68	150 g	13	9
Corn pasta, gluten-free, boiled	78	180 g	42	32
Corn Pops™, breakfast cereal	80	30 g	26	21

* Average

FOOD	GI	NOMINAL SERVE SIZE	AVAILABLE CARB PER SERVE	GL PER SERVE
Corn Thins, puffed corn cakes, gluten-free	87	25 g	20	18
Couscous, boiled 5 min	65*	150 g	33	21
Cranberry juice cocktail	52	250 ml	31	16
Crispix™, breakfast cereal	87	30 g	25	22
Croissant	67	57 g	26	17
Crumpet, white	69	50 g	19	13
Crunchy Nut Cornflakes™ bar	72	30 g	26	19
Crunchy Nut™ Cornflakes	72	30 g	24	17
Cupcake, strawberry-iced	73	38 g	26	19
Custard, home made from milk, (wheat starch), and sugar	43	100 ml	17	7
Custard, prepared from powder with whole milk, No Bake™ (Nestlé)	35	100 ml	17	6
Custard, TRIM™, reduced-fat	37	100 ml	15	6
Custard apple, raw, flesh only	54	120 g	19	10
Dark rye, Blackbread (Riga)	76	30 g	13	10
Dark rye, Schinkenbrot (Riga)	86	30 g	14	12
Dates, dried	103	60 g	40	42
Desiree potato, peeled, boiled 35 min	101	150 g	17	17
Dietworks™ Hazelnut & Apricot bar	42	50 g	22	9
Digestives plain, 2 biscuits	59*	25 g	16	10
Doongara, rice, white, boiled	56*	150 g	42	24
Egg Custard, prepared from powdered mix with whole milk, no bake	35	100 ml	17	6
Eggs	[0]	120 g	0	0
Ensure™, vanilla drink	48	250 ml	34	16

* Average

FOOD	GI	NOMINAL SERVE SIZE	AVAILABLE CARB PER SERVE	GL PER SERVE
Ensure™ bar, chocolate fudge brownie	43	38 g	20	8
Ensure Plus™, vanilla drink	40	237 ml	40	19
Ensure Pudding™, old-fashioned vanilla	36	113 g	26	9
Fanta®, orange soft drink	68	250 ml	34	23
Fettuccine, egg, cooked	32	180 g	46	15
Figs, dried, tenderised	61	60 g	26	16
Fish	[0]	120 g	0	0
Fish fillet, crumbed (Maggi)	43	85 g	16	7
Fish Fingers	38	100 g	19	7
French baguette, white, plain	95	30 g	15	15
French fries, frozen, reheated in microwave	75	150 g	29	22
French vanilla ice-cream, premium, 16% fat (Sara Lee)	38	50 g	9	3
Froot Loops™, breakfast cereal	69	30 g	26	18
Fruche, diet, vanilla	31	200 g	12	4
Frosties™, sugar-coated Cornflakes	55	30 g	26	15
Fruit bites, apple and sultana, Arnott's	45	35 g	25	11
Fructose, pure	19*	10 g	10	2
Vanilla cake made from packet mix with vanilla frosting	42	111 g	58	24
Fruit cocktail, canned (Canada)	55	120 g	16	9
Fruit Fingers, Heinz Kidz™, banana	61	30 g	20	12
Fruit loaf, Bürgen™	44	30 g	13	6
Fruit Loaf, dense continental style wheat bread with dried fruit	47	30 g	15	7
Fruit and Spice Loaf, thick sliced	54	30 g	15	8

* Average

THE NEW GLUCOSE REVOLUTION TABLES

FOOD	GI	NOMINAL SERVE SIZE	AVAILABLE CARB PER SERVE	GL PER SERVE
Gatorade® sports drink	78	250 ml	15	12
Glucodin™ glucose tablets	102	10 g	10	10
Gluten-free white bread, sliced	80	30 g	15	12
Gluten-free multigrain bread	79	30 g	13	10
Gluten-free muesli, with 1.5% fat milk	39	30 g	19	7
Gluten-free corn pasta	78	180 g	42	32
Gluten-free rice and maize pasta	76	180 g	49	37
Gluten-free split pea and soy pasta shells	29	180 g	31	9
Gluten-free spaghetti, rice and split pea, canned in tomato sauce	68	220 g	27	19
Glutinous rice, white, cooked in rice cooker	98	150 g	32	31
Gnocchi, cooked (Latina)	68	180 g	48	33
Golden Wheats™, breakfast cereal	71	30 g	23	16
Grapefruit, raw	25	120 g	11	3
Grapefruit juice, unsweetened	48	250 ml	20	9
Grapes, green	46*	120 g	18	8
Green pea soup, canned	66	250 ml	41	27
Guardian™, breakfast cereal	37	30 g	12	5
Hamburger bun	61	30 g	15	9
Haricot/navy beans, cooked/canned	38*	150 g	31	12
Healthwise™ breakfast cereal for bowel health	66	30 g	18	12
Healthwise™ breakfast cereal for heart health	48	30 g	19	9
Helga's™ Classic Seed Loaf	68	30 g	14	9
Helga's™ traditional wholemeal bread	70	30 g	13	9

* Average

FOOD	GI	NOMINAL SERVE SIZE	AVAILABLE CARB PER SERVE	GL PER SERVE
Honey, Yellow Box honey	35	25 g	18	6
Honey, Stringybark	44	25 g	21	9
Honey, Ironbark	48	25 g	15	7
Honey, Capilano	64*	25 g	17	11
Honey & Oat bread, Vogel's	55	30 g	14	7
Honey Rice Bubbles™, breakfast cereal	77	30 g	27	20
Honey Smacks™, breakfast cereal	71	30 g	23	11
Ice-cream, Norco Prestige Light rich Vanilla	47	50 g	10	5
Ice-cream, Norco Prestige Light Toffee	37	50 g	14	5
Ice-cream, Norco Prestige Macadamia	39	50 g	12	5
Ice-cream, regular, average	61*	50 g	13	8
Ice-cream, Peter's light and creamy	44	100 ml	14	6
Ice-cream, premium, French vanilla, 16% fat	38	50 g	9	3
Ice-cream, premium, 'ultra chocolate', 15% fat	37	50 g	9	4
Instant mashed potato, prepared	69*	150 g	20	17
Instant rice, white, cooked 6 min	87	150 g	42	29
Ironman PR bar®, chocolate	39	65 g	26	10
Isostar® sports drink	70	250 ml	18	13
Jam, apricot fruit spread, reduced sugar	55	30 g	13	7
Jam, strawberry, regular	51	30 g	20	10
Jasmine rice, white, long-grain, cooked in rice cooker	109	150 g	42	46
Jatz™, plain salted cracker biscuits	55	25 g	17	10

* Average

FOOD	GI	NOMINAL SERVE SIZE	AVAILABLE CARB PER SERVE	GL PER SERVE
Jelly Beans	78*	30 g	28	22
Jevity™, fibre-enriched drink	48	237 ml	36	17
Just Right™, breakfast cereal	60	30 g	22	13
Just Right Just Grains™, breakfast cereal	62	30 g	23	14
Kaiser rolls	73	30 g	16	12
Kavli™ Norwegian Crispbread	71	25 g	16	12
Kidney beans, canned	52	150 g	17	9
Kidz™, Heinz, Fruit Fingers, banana	61	30 g	20	12
Kidney beans, boiled	28*	150 g	25	7
Kiwi fruit, raw	58	120 g	12	7
Komplete™, breakfast cereal	48	30 g	21	10
K-Time Just Right™ breakfast cereal bar	72	30 g	24	17
K-Time Strawberry Crunch™ breakfast cereal bar	77	30 g	25	19
Lactose, pure	46*	10 g	10	5
Lamb	[0]	120 g	0	0
Lamingtons, sponge dipped in chocolate and coconut	87	50 g	29	25
L.E.A.N Fibergy™ bar, Harvest Oat	45	50 g	29	13
L.E.A.N Life long Nutribar™, Peanut Crunch	30	40 g	19	6
L.E.A.N Life long Nutribar™, Chocolate Crunch	32	40 g	19	6
L.E.A.N Nutrimeal™, drink powder, Dutch Chocolate	26	250 g	13	3
Lebanese bread, white, 1 round	75	83 g	45	34
Lentils, canned, green	52	50 g	17	9

* Average

FOOD	GI	NOMINAL SERVE SIZE	AVAILABLE CARB PER SERVE	GL PER SERVE
Lentils, green, dried, boiled	30*	150 g	17	5
Lentils, boiled	29*	150 g	18	5
Lentils, red, boiled	26	150 g	18	5
Life Savers®, peppermint	70	30 g	30	21
Light rye bread	68	30 g	14	10
Lima beans, baby, frozen, reheated in microwave oven	32	150 g	30	10
Linguine pasta, thick, cooked	46*	180 g	48	22
Linguine pasta, thin, cooked	52*	180 g	45	23
Lowan honey-toasted breakfast cereal	68	50 g	37	25
Lucozade®, original, sparkling glucose drink	95	250 ml	42	40
Lungkow beanthread noodles	26	180 g	45	12
Lychees, canned in syrup, drained	79	120 g	20	16
M & M's®, peanut	33	30 g	17	6
Macaroni, plain, boiled	47*	180 g	48	23
Macaroni and Cheese, made from mix	64	180 g	51	32
Maltose, 50 g	105	10 g	10	11
Mango raw	51*	120 g	17	8
Maple syrup, Pure Canadian	54	24 g	18	10
Marmalade, orange	48	30 g	20	9
Mars Bar®	62	60 g	40	25
Melba toast	70	30 g	23	16
Milk, full-fat cow's milk, fresh	31	250 ml	12	4
Milk, skim	32	250 ml	13	4
Milk, low fat, chocolate, with sugar, Lite White™	34	250 ml	26	9
Milk, condensed, sweetened	61	50 ml	28	17

* Average

FOOD	GI	NOMINAL SERVE SIZE	AVAILABLE CARB PER SERVE	GL PER SERVE
Milk Arrowroot™ biscuits	69	25 g	18	12
Milky Bar®, plain, white chocolate	44	50 g	29	13
Millet, boiled	71	150 g	36	25
Milo™, chocolate powder, dissolved in water	54	250 ml	16	9
Milo™, ready to drink bottle	30	600 ml	66	20
Mini Wheats™, whole wheat breakfast cereal	58	30 g	21	12
Mini Wheats™, blackcurrant whole wheat breakfast cereal	72	30 g	21	15
Mixed grain loaf, Bürgen®	49*	30 g	11	6
Morning Coffee™, 3 biscuits	79	25 g	19	15
Mousse, butterscotch, reduced fat	36	50 g	10	4
Mousse, chocolate, reduced fat	31	50 g	11	3
Mousse, hazelnut, reduced fat	36	50 g	10	4
Mousse, mango, reduced fat	33	50 g	11	4
Mousse, mixed berry, reduced fat	36	50 g	10	4
Mousse, strawberry, reduced fat	32	50 g	10	3
Muesli bar containing dried fruit	61	30 g	21	13
Muesli, gluten-free with 1.5% fat milk	39	30 g	19	7
Muesli, toasted (Purina)	43	30 g	17	7
Muesli, Swiss Formula, natural	56	30 g	16	9
Multi-Grain 9-Grain	43	30 g	14	6
Mung bean noodles (Lungkow beanthread), dried, boiled	39	180 g	45	18
Naytura, natural muesli	65	60 g	33	21
Nesquik™ powder, chocolate dissolved in 1.5% fat milk	41	250 ml	11	5

* Average

FOOD	GI	NOMINAL SERVE SIZE	AVAILABLE CARB PER SERVE	GL PER SERVE
Nesquik™ powder, strawberry dissolved in 1.5% fat milk	35	250 ml	12	4
New potato, unpeeled and boiled 20 min	78	150 g	21	16
New potato, canned, heated in microwave 3 min	65	150 g	18	12
No Bake Egg Custard, prepared from powder with whole milk	35	100 ml	17	6
Noodles, instant 'two-minute' Maggi®	47*	180 g	40	19
Noodles, mung bean (Lungkow beanthread), dried, boiled	39	180 g	45	18
Noodles, rice, freshly made, boiled	40	180 g	39	15
Norco Ice-cream, Prestige Light rich Vanilla	47	50 g	10	5
Norco Ice-cream, Prestige Light Toffee	37	50 g	14	5
Norco Ice-cream, Prestige Macadamia	39	50 g	12	5
Nutella®, chocolate hazelnut spread	33	20 g	12	4
Nutrigrain™, breakfast cereal	66	30 g	15	10
Oat 'n' Honey Bake™, breakfast cereal	77	30 g	17	13
Oat Bran & Honey Loaf bread, Bürgen®	49	40 g	13	7
Oat bran, raw	55*	10 g	5	3
Orange, 1 medium	42*	120 g	11	5
Orange cordial, reconstituted	66	250 ml	20	13
Orange juice, unsweetened, reconstituted	53	250 ml	18	9
Pancakes, prepared from shake mix	67	70 g	23	15

* Average

FOOD	GI	NOMINAL SERVE SIZE	AVAILABLE CARB PER SERVE	GL PER SERVE
Pancakes, buckwheat, gluten-free, made from packet mix	102	77 g	22	22
Parsnips	97	80 g	12	12
Party pies, beef, cooked	45	100 g	27	12
Pastry, plain	59	57 g	26	15
Paw paw, raw	59*	120 g	8	5
Peach, fresh, 1 large	42*	120 g	11	5
Peach, canned in heavy syrup	58	120 g	15	9
Peach, canned in light syrup	52	120 g	18	9
Peach, canned in reduced-sugar syrup, SPC Lite	62	120 g	17	11
Peanuts, roasted, salted	14*	50 g	6	1
Pear, raw	38*	120 g	11	4
Pear halves, canned in natural juice	43	120 g	13	5
Pear halves, canned in reduced-sugar syrup, (SPC Lite)	25	120 g	14	4
Peas, dried, boiled	22	150 g	9	2
Peas, green, frozen, boiled	48*	80 g	7	3
Pecans (raw)	10	50 g	3	1
Pelde brown rice, boiled	76	150 g	38	29
Performax™ bread	38	30 g	13	5
Pikelets, Golden brand	85	40 g	21	18
Pineapple, raw	59*	120 g	10	6
Pineapple juice, unsweetened	46	250 ml	34	15
Pinto beans, canned in brine	45	150 g	22	10
Pinto beans, dried, boiled	39	150 g	26	10
Pita bread, white	57	30 g	17	10
Pizza, cheese	60	100 g	27	16

* Average

FOOD	GI	NOMINAL SERVE SIZE	AVAILABLE CARB PER SERVE	GL PER SERVE
Pizza, Super Supreme, pan (11.4% fat)	36	100 g	24	9
Pizza, Super Supreme, thin and crispy (13.2 % fat)	30	100 g	22	7
Ploughman's™ Wholegrain bread, original recipe	47	30 g	14	7
Ploughman's™ Wholemeal bread, smooth milled	64	30 g	13	9
Plums, raw	39*	120 g	12	5
Pontiac potato, peeled, boiled 35 min	88	150 g	18	16
Pontiac potato, peeled and microwave on high for 6–7.5 min	79	150 g	18	14
Pontiac potato, peeled, cubed, boiled 15 min, mashed	91	150 g	20	18
Pop Tarts™, Double Chocolate	70	50 g	36	25
Popcorn, plain, cooked in microwave oven	72*	20 g	11	8
Pork	[0]	120 g	0	0
Porridge made from whole oats	55	250 g	21	12
Potato crisps, plain, salted	54*	50 g	21	11
Pound cake	54	53 g	28	15
Poweraid®	65	250 ml	20	13
Power Bar®, chocolate	56*	65 g	42	24
Pretzels, oven-baked, traditional wheat flavour	83	30 g	20	16
Prunes, pitted, 6	29	60 g	33	10
Pudding, instant, chocolate, made from powder and whole milk	47	100 g	16	7
Pudding, instant, vanilla, made from powder and whole milk	40	100 g	16	6

* Average

FOOD	GI	NOMINAL SERVE SIZE	AVAILABLE CARB PER SERVE	GL PER SERVE
Pudding, Sustagen™, instant vanilla, made from powdered mix	27	250 g	47	13
Puffed crispbread	81	25 g	19	15
Puffed rice cakes, white	82	25 g	21	17
Puffed Wheat, breakfast cereal	80	30 g	21	17
Pumpernickel rye kernel bread	50*	30 g	12	6
Pumpkin	75	80 g	4	3
Quik™, chocolate (Nestlé, Australia), dissolved in 1.5% fat milk	41	250 ml	11	5
Quik™, strawberry (Nestlé, Australia), dissolved in 1.5% fat milk	35	250 ml	12	4
Raisins	64	60 g	44	28
Ravioli, durum wheat flour, meat filled, boiled	39	180 g	38	15
Real Fruit Bars, strawberry processed fruit bars	90	30 g	26	23
Rice and maize pasta, Ris'O'Mais, gluten-free	76	180 g	49	37
Rice Bran, extruded	19	30 g	14	3
Rice Bubbles™, breakfast cereal	87	30 g	26	22
Rice Bubble Treat™ bar	63	30 g	24	15
Rice cakes, white	82	25 g	21	17
Rice Krispies™, breakfast cereal	82	30 g	26	22
Rice noodles, freshly made, boiled	40	180 g	39	15
Rice pasta, brown, boiled 16 min	92	180 g	38	35
Rice vermicelli, dried, boiled	58	180 g	39	22
Rich Tea, 2 biscuits	55	25 g	19	10
Risotto rice, arborio, boiled	69	150 g	43	29

* Average

FOOD	GI	NOMINAL SERVE SIZE	AVAILABLE CARB PER SERVE	GL PER SERVE
Rockmelon/cantaloupe, raw	68	165 g	8	5
Roggenbrot, Vogel's	59	30 g	14	8
Roll (bread), Kaiser	73	30 g	16	12
Roll-Ups®, processed fruit snack	99	30 g	25	24
Romano beans	46	150 g	18	8
Rye bread, wholemeal	58*	30 g	14	8
Ryvita™ crackers	69	25 g	16	11
Salami	[0]	120 g	0	0
Salmon	0	150 g	0	0
Sao™, plain square crackers	70	25 g	17	12
Sausages, fried	28	100 g	3	1
Scones, plain, made from packet mix	92	25 g	9	8
Sebago potato, peeled, boiled 35 min	87	150 g	17	14
Semolina cooked	55*	150 g	11	6
Shellfish (prawns, crab, lobster etc)	[0]	120 g	0	0
Shortbread biscuits	64	25 g	16	10
Shredded Wheat, breakfast cereal	75*	30 g	20	15
Shredded Wheatmeal™ biscuits	62	25 g	18	11
Skittles®	70	50 g	45	32
Snack Right Fruit Slice, original, Arnott's	48	35 g	26	12
Snack Right Fruit Roll, spicy apple and sultana, Arnott's	45	35 g	25	11
So Natural™ soy milk, full-fat (3%), 120 mg calcium, Calciforte	36	250 ml	18	6
So Natural™ soy milk, reduced-fat (1.5%), 120 mg calcium, Light	44	250 ml	17	8
So Natural™ soy milk, full-fat (3%), 0 mg calcium, Original	44	250 ml	17	8

* Average

113

FOOD	GI	NOMINAL SERVE SIZE	AVAILABLE CARB PER SERVE	GL PER SERVE
So Natural™ soy smoothie drink, banana, 1% fat	30	250 ml	22	7
So Natural™ soy smoothie drink, chocolate hazelnut, 1% fat	34	250 ml	25	8
So Natural™ soy yoghurt, peach and mango, 2% fat, sugar	50	200 ml	26	13
Sourdough rye	48	30 g	12	6
Sourdough wheat	54	30 g	14	8
Soy milk, So Natural™ full-fat (3%), 120 mg calcium, Calciforte	36	250 ml	18	6
Soy milk, So Natural™ reduced-fat (1.5%), 120 mg calcium, Light	44	250 ml	17	8
Soy milk, So Natural™ full-fat (3%), 0 mg calcium, Original	44	250 ml	17	8
Soy smoothie drink, So Natural™ banana, 1% fat	30	250 ml	22	7
Soy smoothie drink, So Natural™ chocolate hazelnut, 1% fat	34	250 ml	25	8
Soy yoghurt, So Natural™ peach and mango, 2% fat, sugar	50	200 g	26	13
Soy beans, dried, boiled	18*	150 g	6	1
Soy beans, canned	14	150 g	6	1
Soy-Lin, Bürgen® kibbled soy (8%) and linseed (8%) bread	36	30 g	9	3
Spaghetti, gluten-free, rice and split pea, canned in tomato sauce	68	220 g	27	19
Spaghetti, white, boiled 5 minutes	38*	180 g	48	18
Spaghetti, wholemeal, boiled 5 minutes	37	180 g	42	16
Special K®, breakfast cereal	54	30 g	21	11

* Average

FOOD	GI	NOMINAL SERVE SIZE	AVAILABLE CARB PER SERVE	GL PER SERVE
Spirali pasta, durum wheat, white, boiled to al denté texture	43	180 g	44	19
Split pea and soy pasta shells, gluten-free	29	180 g	31	9
Split pea soup	60	250 ml	27	16
Split peas, yellow, boiled 20 min	32	150 g	19	6
Sponge cake, plain	46	63 g	36	17
Stoned Wheat Thins crackers	67	25 g	17	12
Strawberries, fresh	40	120 g	3	1
Strawberry jam, regular	51	30 g	20	10
Stuffing, bread	74	30 g	21	16
Sucrose	68*	10 g	10	7
Sultana Bran™, breakfast cereal	73	30 g	19	14
Sultanas	56	60 g	45	25
Sunbrown Quick™ rice, boiled	80	150 g	38	31
Sunflower and barley bread, (Riga)	57	30 g	11	6
Super Supreme pizza, pan (11.4% fat)	36	100 g	24	9
Super Supreme pizza, thin and crispy (13.2 % fat)	30	100 g	22	7
Sushi, salmon	48	100 g	36	17
Sustagen™ Hospital with extra fibre, drink made from powdered mix	33	250 ml	44	15
Sustagen™ drink, Dutch Chocolate	31	250 ml	41	13
Sustagen™ pudding, instant vanilla, made from powdered mix	27	250 ml	47	13
Sustagen Sport®, milk-based drink	43	250 ml	49	21
Sustain™, breakfast cereal	68	30 g	22	15
Sustain™ cereal bar	57	30 g	25	14
Swede, cooked	72	150 g	10	7

* Average

FOOD	GI	NOMINAL SERVE SIZE	AVAILABLE CARB PER SERVE	GL PER SERVE
Sweet corn, whole kernel, canned, drained	46	80 g	14	7
Sweet corn on the cob, boiled	48	80 g	16	8
Sweet potato, cooked	44	150 g	25	11
Sweetened condensed whole milk	61	50 g	28	17
Taco shells, cornmeal-based, baked	68	20 g	12	8
Tapioca, boiled with milk	81	250 ml	18	14
Tomato soup	38	250 ml	17	6
Tortellini, cheese, cooked	50	180 g	21	10
TRIM™ custard, reduced-fat	37	100 g	15	6
Tuna	[0]	120 g	0	0
Twisties™, cheese-flavoured, extruded snack, rice and corn	74	50 g	29	22
Twix® Bar, caramel	44	60 g	39	17
Ultra chocolate ice-cream, premium 15% fat (Sara Lee)	37	50 g	9	4
Vaalia™, reduced-fat apricot and mango yoghurt	26	200 g	30	8
Vaalia™, reduced-fat French vanilla yoghurt	26	200 g	10	3
Vaalia™, reduced fat tropical passionfruit yoghurt drink	38	200 ml	29	11
Vanilla cake made from packet mix with vanilla frosting	42	111 g	58	24
Vanilla pudding, instant, made from packet mix and whole milk	40	100 g	16	6
Vanilla wafers, 6 biscuits	77	25 g	18	14
Veal	[0]	120 g	0	0
Vermicelli, white, boiled	35	180 g	44	16

* Average

FOOD	GI	NOMINAL SERVE SIZE	AVAILABLE CARB PER SERVE	GL PER SERVE
Vita-Brits™, breakfast cereal	68	30 g	20	13
Vita Weat crispbread	55	35 g	26	14
Vitari, wild berry, non-dairy, frozen fruit dessert	59	100 ml	21	12
Vogel's Honey & Oats bread	55	30 g	14	7
Waffles	76	35 g	13	10
Water crackers	78	25 g	18	14
Watermelon, raw	76	195 g	10	7
Weis Mango Frutia™, low fat frozen fruit dessert	42	100 ml	23	10
Weet-Bix™, breakfast cereal	69	30 g	17	12
Wheat-bites™, breakfast cereal	72	30 g	25	18
White bread, wheat flour	70	30 g	14	10
Wholemeal bread, wheat flour	71*	30 g	12	9
Wild About Fruit Apple Juice, pure, clear, unsweetened	44	250 ml	30	13
Wild About Fruit Apple Juice, pure, cloudy, unsweetened	37	250 ml	28	10
Wild About Fruit Apple and mandarin juice	53	250 ml	29	15
Wild About Fruit Apple and mango juice	44	250 ml	27	12
Wonderwhite™ bread	80	30 g	14	11
Yam, peeled, boiled	37*	150 g	36	13
Yoghurt, diet, low fat, no added sugar, vanilla	23	200 g	13	3
Yoghurt, diet, low fat, no added sugar, (fruit)	24*	200 g	13	3
Yoghurt drink, Vaalia™, reduced-fat tropical passionfruit	38	200 ml	29	11

* Average

FOOD	GI	NOMINAL SERVE SIZE	AVAILABLE CARB PER SERVE	GL PER SERVE
Yoghurt, low fat, fruit with artificial sweetener	14	200 g	13	2
Yoghurt, low fat, fruit with sugar	33	200 g	31	10
Yoghurt, low fat (0.9%), wild strawberry	31	200 g	30	9
Yoghurt, low fat, sugar sweetened, strawberry, Yoplait	33	200 g	31	10
Yoghurt, no-fat, French vanilla, Vaalia, with sugar	40	150 g	27	10
Yoghurt, no-fat, Mango, Vaalia, with sugar	39	150 g	25	10
Yoghurt, no-fat, strawberry, sweetened, Yoplait	19	200 g	13	2
Yoghurt, no-fat, Strawberry, Vaalia, with sugar	38	150 g	22	8
Yoghurt, no-fat, Wildberry, Vaalia, with sugar	38	150 g	22	8
Yoplait BFast breakfast drink, honey banana malt	33	250 ml	27	9

* Average

How to find a sports dietitan

The best way to obtain the names of sport dietitians practising in your area is to contact:

Sports Dietitians Australia
Level 8, Victorian Institute of Sport
20-22 Albert Road, South Melbourne
PO Box 828, South Melbourne, 3205
Telephone (03) 9682 2442
Fax (03) 9686 2352

It is also worth checking in the *Yellow Pages* for your area.

Most state institutes of sport have sports dietitians consulting with their athletes.

ASDA (Australian Sports Drug Agency)
PO Box 345
Curtin ACT 2605
Australia
Phone: +61 (0)2 6206 0200
Fax: +61 (0)2 6206 0201
www.asda.org.au

Recommended reading on sports nutrition

For an expanded discussion on sports nutrition the following books are highly recommended:

Burke L. (1995), *The Complete Guide to Food for Sports Performance*, London, Allen and Unwin

Cardwell G. (1996), *Gold Medal Nutrition*, Glenn Cardwell (self published)

Garden L. (1993), *Footy Food*, Lorna Garden (self published)

O'Connor H and Hay D. (1993), *The Taste of Fitness*, Sydney, NSW, JB Fairfax Press

Roberts C and Inge K. (1993), *Food for Sport Cookbook*, Abbotsford, Vic, Rene Gordon

About the authors

Dr Helen O'Connor is a sports dietitian and lecturer in the Department of Exercise and Sport Science at the University of Sydney. Helen consults at the Sydney Sports Medicine Centre, Olympic Park, and at South Sydney Sports Medicine Centre. She is a consultant dietitian to the Sydney Swans, Canterbury Rugby League and a number of Australia's elite athletes.

Professor Jennie Brand-Miller is a Professor of Human Nutrition in the Human Nutrition Unit at the University of Sydney and President of the Nutrition Society of Australia. Professor Brand-Miller was awarded the prestigious Clunies Ross National Science and Technology Medal for her work on nutrition and the management of blood sugar.

Professor Stephen Colagiuri, Director of the Diabetes Centre and Head of the Department of Endocrinology, Metabolism and Diabetes at the Prince of Wales Hospital, Sydney, has published extensively on carbohydrate in the diet of people with diabetes.

Kaye Foster-Powell is an accredited practising dietitian with extensive experience in diabetes management. She has conducted research into the glycemic index of foods and its practical applications over the last 15 years. Currently she is a dietitian with Wentworth Area Diabetes Services and provides consultancy on all aspects of the glycemic index.